SENIOR FITNESS

Balance and Strength Training

Using Light Weights

RON KNESS

Contents

Disclaimer

Use caution when beginning a new wellness program. Not all exercise programs are suitable for everyone. Check with your doctor before you begin.

Ron Kness will not be responsible or liable for any injury sustained as a result of using any program presented and/or discussed on his blog, via this book, email communications or in video format.

Introduction

As we age, most people notice a range of changes in their health. I know I have in mine. One change might not seem like such a big deal, but more than one can add up to poor health long-term. For example, we might notice we are not as strong as we once were.

We might discover that our balance isn't what it used to be. It takes me a couple of minutes now in the morning after I first get up to get my balance in check. I usually bounce off of the hallway walls a couple of times at least on my way to the kitchen to make coffee. As a result we may be prone to losing our balance and injuring ourselves due to slips, trips and falls.

With aging comes a number of illnesses that can affect our fitness and mobility, such as arthritis and osteoporosis. We might also suffered from heart or lung disorders which can affect our stamina and endurance. These conditions might all seem to limit our ability to exercise, leading people to believe they can't or shouldn't work out.

In fact, nothing could be further from the truth. Exercising, including strength training, can help relieve the symptoms of many of these conditions, easing pain and stiffness and helping your heart and lungs work more efficiently, thus improving your overall health. My doctor told me the best way to deal with my osteoarthritis is to keep moving. So far it is working the best of anything I have tried.

Many older people shy away from exercise because they fear pain or injury. They might also think they have to spend hours in a gym working out to see any results, so why bother. Women in particular might hate the idea of pumping iron or sweating buckets.

They might even feel embarrassed going to a gym that is full of young, healthy 20-somethings who are built like twigs.

The truth is that working out with light weights is easy to do at home. You can get results in as few as 10 minutes a day, often without even breaking a sweat.

If you do decide to exercise with a workout partner, this can also lead to emotional health and well-being.

In this guide, we will outline the benefits of light weights for your health, balance and strength, and how to get started using light weights safely and inexpensively. Let's start with how light weights can help your joints.

Chapter 1 – How Light Weights Can Improve Joint Health

As we age, the wear and tear on our joints from a lifetime of activity can start to take its toll in the form of osteoarthritis (OA) (http://www.arthritis.org/about-arthritis/types/osteoarthritis/). OA is common from middle age onwards and is the result of the joint cartilage and the bone underneath it wearing out over time. The most common symptoms of OA are pain and stiffness in the joints, particularly the hips, knees and hands. The pain and stiffness from OA makes sufferers shy away from exercising. The truth is that inactivity can lead to even more stiffness.

The best exercises for those with OA are low impact ones, including working out with light weights. Other safe and sensible choices are walking, yoga, tai chi, swimming, and water aerobics. Light weights can easily be worked into even the busiest of schedules. Best of all, you can use them in the convenience of your own home.

Many women in particular also develop rheumatoid arthritis (RA) (http://www.arthritis.org/about-arthritis/types/rheumatoid-arthritis/what-is-rheumatoid-arthritis.php) as they get older. RA is an autoimmune disorder, that is, a condition which is caused by the body attacking itself. No one is sure exactly why this happens, but the results are clear. RA damages the joints and can lead to painful deformities (gnarled-looking joints), especially in the hands, wrists, elbows, knees and ankles.

One of the best ways to relieve the pain and damage of RA is to exercise regularly, (http://www.webmd.com/rheumatoid-arthritis/guide/exercise-and-rheumatoid-arthritis) in a number of ways.

(http://www.webmd.com/rheumatoid-arthritis/patient-support-12/slideshow-ra-exercises).

Lifting heavy weights can cause further damage to joints, but light weights can improve mobility and prevent the thinning of the bones that often occurs with RA. Let's look in the next chapter at how light weights can improve bone health.

Chapter 2 – How Light Weights Can Improve Bone Strength

Most people think their bones are solid and unchanging. In reality, our bones are constantly being broken down and built back up again. In order to maintain bone health, you need to eat a balanced diet rich in nutrients such as calcium and Vitamin D. Weight bearing exercise is also essential in order to avoid two common conditions that lead to thinning of the bone, osteopenia and osteoporosis.

If we think of healthy bone as a brick wall with 100 bricks, osteopenia would result in a wall with only 90 or 80 bricks, and osteoporosis in a wall with only 70 or 60 bricks. This leaves the bones more prone to breaking, especially if an older person trips and falls. Falling is the number one thing that causes injuries in older adults.

These conditions also leave you more prone to injury due to jagged and rough bone formation, such as bone spurs. Bone spurs can pinch nerves or result in the 'snap, crackle and pop' we associate with old age (crepitus), caused by tendons stretching over bones and joints.

Changes in bone formation can also lead to spinal stenosis, in which the bones of the vertebrae in your spine begin to narrow and can pinch your nerves. This can result in nerve damage, back pain, numbness and/or a loss of mobility due to the pain causing people to avoid physical activity and thus get even stiffer.

Avoiding exercise due to the pain will only lead to even more pain and stiffness, a vicious cycle that will ruin your quality of life unless you decide to start working out more regularly. Light weights help build strong, healthy bones by boosting bone mass.

Since women tend to lose bone rapidly after menopause, they can benefit most from light weights, push-ups, and exercises such as brisk walking and yoga. A bone density test can help you determine whether or not you have osteopenia or osteoporosis and what the most effective treatments will be for your condition. Your doctor will certainly recommend weight-bearing exercise as part of your treatment.

Squats, step-ups and lunges are all good for improving bone density. These can be done using light weights in your hands, or a medicine ball if you prefer, and an aerobics step or the bottom stair of your staircase if you have one. A staircase works good because the rail give you something to grab if you feel you are going to fall or start falling.

Another way to protect your bones is to improve your balance, strength and stability in order to avoid injuries which can lead to fractures. Let's look at how light weights can improve your balance, strength and stability in the next chapter.

Chapter 3 – How Light Weights Can Improve Your Balance, Strength and Stability

Light weight workouts are not just beneficial for your joints and bones. They can also help you improve the balance, strength and the stability of your joints. All of these are important in order to avoid injuries such as falls, which are common in older people. They are dangerous because they can lead to broken bones such as a fractured hip. Broken bones of any kind can mean loss of mobility both short- and long-term and other potentially dangerous complications as well, such as blood clots in the legs or pneumonia due to inactivity. Some people never do fully recover from a broken hip and end up in an assisted care facility or nursing home.

In terms of strength, most people think that they have to pump iron and do endless repetitions with heavy weights to see results. However, an increasing number of studies have shown that consistent effort with light weights is just as effective as heavy weights. The only reason for using heavier weights is if your goal is to get large muscles – extremely difficult for anyone over 50. If you just want to stay toned and trim, light weights will be more than enough.

In relation to balance, tai chi and yoga can help boost balance. Add light hand, wrist and/or ankle weights to your yoga or tai chi moves as appropriate in order to improve balance as well as strength. Another option is to alternate one side of the body or the other, standing on one foot while lifting weights and then switching sides.

If you are trying to get a full body workout of arms, core and legs, use wrist and/or ankle weights. For example, start on your hands and knees and extend your right arm out in front of you and your left leg behind you, trying to maintain a straight line – called the bird dog by the way in yoga. Then repeat the exercise in the opposite manner, stretching out your left arm in front of you and your right leg behind you. It may be difficult at first, but you will soon see results in a leaner and more toned body.

In terms of stability, training both sides of your body leads to better balance and muscle tone, which in turn increase the stability of your joints. This can maintain mobility if you have either OA or RA and prevent further damage or injury.

Light weights are not just good for your bones, muscles and joints. In the next chapter we will discuss how light weights can improve your circulation, lower cholesterol, and improve your blood glucose levels.

The most important muscle in your body is your heart. Light weights can improve your heart health by working it to keep it strong. Light weights combined with cardio have been shown to help relieve or manage a range of cardiovascular conditions (http://circ.ahajournals.org/content/101/7/828.full) even in low to moderate risk heart patients. Working out even a few minutes a day can reduce the likelihood of a heart attack and improve quality of life by relieving depression, which heart patients and those with other chronic conditions such as arthritis or diabetes often experience.

Light weights have been shown to lower blood pressure; however, heavier weights appear to increase it. This is most likely due to the strain of lifting such heavy weights.

Therefore, if you already have high blood pressure, be sure to check with your doctor before undertaking any weight training exercises.

Lifting light weights improves your circulation. Better circulation will usually mean lower blood pressure, lower cholesterol and more rapid elimination of waste and toxins from your body. When your blood pressure and cholesterol are low, you are much less likely to suffer from cardiovascular issues, heart attack, or stroke.

With so many people in the US and around the world overweight or obese, they are at increased risk of heart health issues. In particular, those with rheumatoid arthritis are especially prone to cardiovascular problems.

For those who are overweight or obese, many of them might also be prediabetes or diabetic and not even know it. Many people with diabetes also have heart issues.

Type 2 diabetes has become almost an epidemic amongst older adults. A study published in September 2015 estimates that diabetes and prediabetes now affect 50% of the US population, with many unaware that they have it, and that it is particularly common amongst certain ethnicities.

With diabetes, the pancreas is not able to produce enough of the hormone insulin, which results in elevated sugar (glucose) in the blood. Diabetes that is not kept under control can lead to a range of health issues, such as high or low blood sugar that can lead to serious illness or even death. Diabetes can also result in damage to the eyes (diabetic retinopathy), the kidneys, (diabetic nephropathy) and nerves, such as the nerves in the hands (diabetic neuropathy).

Diabetes is also the #2 cause of amputation, after accidents, most often affecting the toes, feet and legs. This can lead to a lack of mobility and loss of wages, productivity and quality of life.

It can also make it very difficult to exercise or even just perform the usual activities of daily life such as bathing, shopping and cooking.

Fortunately, many light weights workouts can be performed sitting or lying down, not just standing up.

One other major health concern related to cardiovascular issues is known as metabolic syndrome. This is a cluster of abnormal health readings that also appear to signal the likelihood of the person developing Type 2 diabetes or experiencing a major event such as a heart attack or stroke.

Metabolic syndrome is diagnosed on the basis of a person having 3 out of the following 5 symptoms:

1. **high blood pressure**

2. **high blood glucose levels**

3. **a high level of visceral fat, or waist roundness (a spare tire)**

4. **low levels of good cholesterol, that is, HDL cholesterol (think H for helpful)**

5. **high triglycerides on your cholesterol test**

Triglycerides are a type of fat found in your blood which circulates energy throughout your body to make it available for all the activities you do throughout the day. However, if you do not have a very active lifestyle, the triglycerides will be stored in your fat cells. Hormones release the triglycerides for energy between meals. If you regularly eat more calories than you burn, especially calories from carbohydrates (carbs) and unhealthy fats, you can develop high triglycerides (hypertriglyceridemia).

Experts are not sure how high triglycerides contribute to hardening of the arteries or thickening of the artery walls (arteriosclerosis), but we do know arteriosclerosis increases the risk of stroke, heart attack and heart disease.

Extremely high triglycerides can also cause acute pancreatitis. The pancreas is important for digestion and the production of insulin. Many people with metabolic syndrome have insulin resistance-that is, their body produces insulin but the body does not respond to it as it should. This can lead to issues with your metabolism, making it hard to lose weight.

6-Being overweight

While not listed as a specific symptom of metabolic syndrome, people who have any of the five symptoms we have discussed above usually tend to be overweight and out of shape.

While metabolic syndrome might sound terrible, and it can be dangerous, the good news is that exercise can help reduce your risks of heart disease and diabetes even in as little as 150 minutes a week, about 20 minutes a day. This is the current Centers for Disease Control and Prevention (CDC) recommendation for physical activity for adults in order to maintain health. They also suggest strength training twice a week for all adults.

Strength training in particular can be a valuable part of reversing metabolic syndrome and losing weight. This is because of its effects upon the metabolism. Let's look at this topic in more detail in the next chapter.

Chapter 5 – How Light Weights Can Improve Your Metabolism

In the last chapter we discussed how light weights can improve your circulation and blood glucose levels, lower cholesterol and lessen the group of symptoms commonly referred to as metabolic syndrome.

As the name suggests, metabolic syndrome affects the metabolism of your body. Think of metabolism as the engine of our car. The food we eat is the fuel for the engine. Are we giving it high quality or low quality fuel?

Experts can tune an engine to improve its performance, such as more power and better gas mileage. In the same way, our metabolism helps determine our body's performance in relation to how it uses the fuel we consume.

Our metabolism is responsible for whether or not the energy from the food we eat will be released for use by the body right away, or stored in our tissues such as the liver, muscles, and body fat in order to be used later.

Our metabolism is a delicate balancing act influenced greatly by insulin, which we have already mentioned, and thyroid hormones (thyroxine). Low insulin and thyroxine will slow down your metabolism, meaning too much storage of energy and not enough burning of energy, leading to weight gain.

Working out with light weights can boost your metabolism and burn calories more efficiently in a number of ways. First is the movement itself. Any physical movement will burn calories, even sitting. The only difference is the rate at which the calories are burned. Exercise can be as simple as cleaning around the house or lifting light weights. More active whole body exercises include walking, jogging, swimming, or playing tennis. The more vigorous the sport, the more calories burned.

However, as we age, we are less likely to exercise vigorously. High impact activities like jogging, tennis or racquet ball are really not suitable for aging bones and joints. If you use your light weights correctly, there is little risk of injury but great potential benefit to your metabolism.

Remember what we said about the finely tuned engine working more efficiently? Lean muscle in the body burns more calories than fatty tissues in the body. Therefore, strength training that gives you firmer arms, legs and abs can transform your body into a lean, mean, calorie burning machine.

Lifting even light weights can burn 200 calories per 20 minute session depending on tempo and rest breaks. The muscle you develop will boost your natural metabolism and speed up the rate at which you burn your calories. Lowering your calorie consumption to 1600 or 1200 calories and making every calorie count in terms of nutrition, such as through a high protein, low carb diet, can also boost your metabolism. Protein builds more muscle, and more muscle speeds up your metabolism further.

Now that we understand the link between our metabolism and how we use the calories from the food we eat to power our bodies, let's look at how using light weights can help with our weight loss goals and overall physical appearance.

Chapter 6 – How Light Weights Can Help You Lose Weight And Improve Your Appearance

Which take up more space, a pound of cotton balls or a pound of brick? And which is more plump and rounded? In both cases, the answer is cotton balls. Our body without toned muscle is like a group of cotton balls, taking up a lot of space and looking bumpy instead of tight, sleek and smooth.

Cellulite is a good illustration of this. The reason for the 'orange peel' appearance is that the fatty tissues under the skin actually start to poke through our layer of muscle under the skin, thrusting right through to the surface in unsightly bulges. Cellulite can affect belly, butt, thighs and upper arms and lead to negative feelings about one's appearance which in turn can lead to a lack of self-confidence and even depression.

When people first start to use light weights, they may become frustrated because they do not see the scale go down as much as they had hoped. Size-wise muscle weighs more than fat which is one reason why you may not see much of a change on the scale.

You are sculpting those cotton balls into tight, firm muscle so it starts to resemble a brick. The scale may not shift but you will most likely notice that your clothes start to fit better and you look nicer in them. You might even consider going down a size or making your belt tighter as everything starts to firm up.

The best thing about light weights is that you don't just have to use them for a full body workout, although they are ideal for that. Light weights also allow you to focus on your personal trouble spots to enhance your appearance and help you get a 'bikini body' or at least make you feel less self-conscious about wearing shorts, short-sleeved shirts, or tank tops.

Many women hate the flabby chicken wing arms that seem to come with middle age. Men long for six pack abs, not a gut that sticks so far out that they look pregnant. Women also worry about their butt or thighs being too big. Light weights can even help slim down these areas as well if you know which exercises work best for which trouble zones.

If you are tired of tight clothes or jiggling like jelly in them, it's time to look at both calorie consumption and calorie burning, and the best ways to use light weights to target your problem areas.

We are what we eat. The Mayo Clinic has a range of suggested food pyramids (http://www.mayoclinic.org/healthy-lifestyle/nutrition-and-healthy-eating/in-depth/healthy-weight-pyramid/art-20045416) depending on your eating lifestyle, such as being vegetarian or wishing to follow the Mediterranean diet. Use these guidelines to help get your eating back on track so you will eat more healthily.

Use a good food database (http://nutritiondata.self.com/) to count calories and/or carbs. Gradually increase your level of activity, aerobics (cardio) one day, strength training with your light weights the next, and you will soon start to see results as you transform yourself into a trim, toned, more confident you.

If you are still sitting on the fence about whether or not light weights are right for you, chances are it is because you might believe some of the common myths about using light weights.

Let's debunk a few of the most common myths in the next chapter.

Chapter 7 – Eight Weight Training Myths That Hold People Bck From Starting Working Out With Light Weights

Even though we know exercise is good for us, there are a number of myths that hold many people back, especially women and seniors, from starting a strength training program. Here are a few myths we would like to explode once and for all so you can improve your health.

Myth 1-I'm too old to lift weights.

Anyone any age can lift weights provided that they pay attention to safety first. In fact, light weights are perfect for anyone over 40. In particular, they can offer great benefit to women who are approaching or going through menopause. They are also excellent for anyone with osteoarthritis, rheumatoid arthritis or osteoporosis, which all usually come when people, in particular women, reach middle age.

Myth 2-I don't have money for an expensive gym membership.

There's no need to go to a gym. You can use your light weights at home, in almost any room of the house and at any time you wish, even while you are watching TV.

Myth 3-Weight machines are the only way to develop strong muscles.

This is also false. Light weights can be far better for developing strong muscles because you work with them in a natural way, creating more muscle activity and therefore toning and strengthening faster.

Resistance bands are another form of weight-bearing exercise that you can use in conjunction with light hand-held weights to work all your muscles in the same way (or even better) than those huge, expensive machines.

4-I don't have a lot of money or room for all sorts of weight lifting equipment.

There's no need to spend a lot on equipment. You can use a range of items you already have in your house to get started, such as cans of food and bottles of liquid from your kitchen or laundry room.

Once you have reached a point where you need to graduate to heavier weights, consider using highly portable and convenient resistance bands or invest in some ankle weights, wrist weights, or dumbbells. Dumbbells will often come in sets on a tower for easy and compact storage. Aquabells are even more convenient, allowing you to adjust them from 2 pounds up to 16 pounds per side. Plus they are portable. Just empty the water and pack them in your suitcase. Fill them once again at your destination and start working out once more.

Myth 5-If I take a break from lifting weights, my muscles will turn back into fat.

This is impossible in both ways. Muscle is not fat, and fat is not muscle. They are two different kinds of tissue. Therefore, it is impossible for muscle to turn into fat. It will lose tone over time, but not in the space of only a couple of days.

Myth 6-I have to lift weights every day to get results.

Since it takes 24 to 48 hours for your muscles to rest and rejuvenate after a workout with light weights, you should only lift every other day at most.

Anything more than that can irritate muscles and cause damage.

Myth 7-Weight lifting will hurt my joints and make my arthritis even worse.

Also not true. One study has shown that people who start and kept up with a strength training program improved their OA of the knee. For those with RA, exercise is essential. Strength training can improve the stability of the joints and lead to less damage from the bone separating or grinding together because they have lost their cartilage that acts as a shock absorber.

Myth 8-I will appear unfeminine and mannish if I lift weights-I don't want bulky muscles like Arnold Schwarzenegger.

Lifting light weights will trim and tone your muscles. Only extremely heavy weights will start to bulk them up noticeably.

There is nothing sexier than a healthy, confident woman. One with toned muscles will certainly be more attractive than an obese woman who does not work out because she is worried about 'bulking up'. Remember the cotton ball to brick comparison and you will soon see how great you can look in your clothes with the help of light weights workouts giving you lean, tight muscles instead of unsightly flab and cellulite.

Chapter 8 – Lifestyle Changes That Can Maximize Your Light Weight Workouts

Working out with light weight can certainly help tone and trim your body and even enable you to lose weight, but exercise alone will not be enough to improve your health and appearance. For example, as you age, skin that has been stretched through being significantly overweight might not bounce back 100%. Even if it does, you need to maintain it through your weight lifting workouts and improve other health-related habits in order to get the most from your workouts. Here are several ways you can improve results:

- Stop smoking

- Avoid alcohol

- Get a good night's sleep; 6-8 hours

- Don't work out 30 minutes before bed time

- Set a regular bed time and stick to it

- Listen to your body with respect to any health conditions you may have

- Short versus long sessions – even 10 minutes a couple of times a day can make a real difference

- Slow versus natural lifting – use slow lifting if you have any joint issues that would be aggravated by a lot of repetitions

- Pay attention to your diet and eating patterns:

➢ Opt for more whole foods and cut out the processed food

➢ Eat on schedule

➢ Count calories

➢ Avoid excessive snacking

➢ Practice portion control

➢ Don't skip breakfast

➢ Add more protein to your diet

Now that you have discovered all the health benefits of strength training using light weights, plus how a few small lifestyle changes can all lead up to big results, let's look next at how to get equipment without spending a fortune.

Chapter 9 – Inexpensive Equipment To Help You Get Started With Your Weight Training

If you have been shying away from beginning a light weights strength training program because you do not have a lot of spare cash, the good news is that you don't need a lot of expensive equipment to get started. The trick is to work with what you already have. Head to the kitchen cupboards to see what cans and bottles you can hold easily. Make sure they are in pairs. Rank them from lightest to heaviest. Liquids will be a lot heavier than you think.

Can't grip them easily due to hand arthritis? Put them in plastic bags and lift with the handles. Wrap a washcloth or tea towel around the handles to stop them from digging into your hands.

Start slowly and increase your repetitions from 8 to 12 to 16 for example to form 1 set. Gradually increase the number of sets you do. Once you are lifting 3 sets of 12 to 16 repetitions easily using what you have in your kitchen cabinet, it might be time to consider getting your own set of weights. You can buy many items second hand online.

As we have mentioned, Aquabells (http://amzn.to/1QLyROn) are very useful because you can fill them with water as needed to gradually increase the weight up to 16 pounds on each side. This means they can grow with you in a way that sets of dumbbells each of a particular weight will not be able to in the long term.

Another excellent choice that will grow with you as your strength grows are resistance bands (http://amzn.to/21xKtX0).

Sets come with a range of band loads, starting at 2 to 4 pounds and increasing to 25 to 30 pounds. Want to increase your loads to your own particular increments? Put more bands on the handle to 'stack' them to increase the weight. A basic set with 5 bands of different loads can actually take you as high as 75 pounds if you stack all of the bands at the same time.

Aquabells and resistance bands are better than regular dumbbells because you can pack them when you travel without worrying about overweight or excess baggage charges. Tuck them safely in their carrying cases and go.

Hand weights can be used in a range of positions and in conjunction with other fitness moves such as squats and lunges. Hand and wrist weights are ideal for targeting arm strength, especially the upper arms.

If you want to focus on your legs, you might wish to consider investing in a pair of ankle weights. They come in a range of styles, from Aquabells to ones that slip over your ankles or shoes, to more heavy duty ones such as the Weider range of products. Go into a sporting goods store to check which feel right for you in terms of comfort and weight.

The Aquabells ankle weights are not a good option, in our opinion, because the straps are not long enough to secure them to your ankle if you try to fill them all the way. However, there are good sets with 1 pound weighted bars in them so you can work your way up from 1 pound to 10, for example, as you progress in strength, such as the All Pro range of weights.(http://amzn.to/21xKzxV)

Your only other essential equipment will be some comfortable clothes that will not chafe with repeated motions, and a good pair of sneakers to offer you support and ensure you do not slip with you are lifting.

You can also lift light weights sitting down. If you wish to do so, ensure you are on a comfortable chair that will not slip around. If you are in a wheelchair, be sure to lock the wheels before each workout.

Now that you know how little it takes to get started, you might be really excited to begin lifting light weights. But hold on a little while longer. In the next chapter, you will find some important safety tips to keep in mind when lifting weights.

Chapter 10 – Putting Safety First When Starting To Use Light Weights

As with any exercise and new workout routine, it is important to assess where you are in terms of your health and fitness so you do not overdo things and become injured. Every exercise carries with it some potential risk of injury, so make staying safe a priority.

1-Pay attention to any underlying medical conditions you might have. Check with your doctor to be sure you are well enough to use light weights.

2-Always warm up before each session. Walking, walk in place, jumping jacks or a light jog in place is better than stretching. Shocking! These activities get your cardio engaged, blood flowing and loosen joints much better than stretching isolated areas.

3-Start slowly-avoid weights that are too heavy.

4-Start slowly-don't overdo it on the repetitions when you are first beginning.

5-Be careful when handling weights so you do not drop them on the floor or your foot, or bang arms and shoulders with them.

6-Alternate muscle groups during each work out session, arms, legs, core, back to arms, and so on.

7-Work out in front of a mirror to make sure you are maintaining correct form. This will help prevent injury.

8-Try slow lifting as well as natural pace lifting. This will cause less wear and tear on your joints than lots of rapid repetitions.

9-Don't forget to cool down at the end of each session. Post exercise stretching improves flexibility and reduces soreness.

10-If you feel pain, stop right away.

Now that you are aware of the most important safety considerations when it comes to using light weights, let's look at several of the most effective exercises to target trouble spots and also give you a good general workout.

Chapter 11 – Light Weights To Target Muscle Groups

 In this chapter we will be discussing a number of exercises which can help you not only get a good full body workout, but also target muscle groups you may wish to focus on in order to improve your strength and/or appearance.

Instead of focusing on a specific area it's important to use an exercise routine that provides systematic and consistent exercise regime for the entire body. Going after "trouble spots" rarely works because you need to address more than a single muscle group.

For example, doing a thousand sit-ups won't result in a flat belly. However, working consistently the core muscle groups will result in a more defined and stronger set of abs, obliques and back muscles. In terms of particular areas, we have grouped the exercises in the following manner.

1) **Arms**
   a. Bicep curls
   b. Reverse bicep curls
   c. Lateral raises
   d. Lateral to overhead raises

2) **Chest and Shoulders**
   a. Pull up
   b. Gorilla lift
   c. Chest presses

3) **Core Strength, Arms and Legs**
   a. Overhead lift
   b. Overhead pull down
   c. Squat Lift

d. Tricep kickbacks with squat

4) Legs
a. Lift and lunge
b. Side extensions
c. Backward extensions
d. Hip and leg extensions

Our choice has been based on exercises that will benefit you in more than one area so you can be certain you are toning all of your muscles. Most of these exercises will be performed with hand held weights (Aquabells), but we have also given you some with wrist or ankle weights using a set of All Pro (10 lb).

Let's start with a dynamic movements to loosen your muscles. Then we will begin with arm exercises to get rid of flabby chicken wing arms and define your biceps and shoulders. When I could find it, I included a representative YouTube video to show you how to do the exercise along with the instructions.

1.) Arm Exercises

Bicep curls
https://www.youtube.com/watch?v=E6VMg0E9JpE

This is probably familiar to most people whenever they think about lifting weights. The important thing with this exercise is to prevent your arm, elbow or wrist from wobbling as you work out. This exercise is done using wrists weights.

- Start standing with the weights resting thigh level, palms facing upwards.

- Lift the weights to shoulder height by bending the elbows until the weights are shoulder height.

- Lower the weights back down to the starting position in a controlled manner.

- Repeat Steps 7 more times, for 1 set of 8.

Gradually increase both the repetitions (up to 16) and the number of sets (such as 3), until you no longer feel the muscle tension. In this case, you will be ready for a heavier weight. Once moved to the heavier weight drop back on the number of repetitions per set and gradually build up again.

Reverse bicep curls
https://www.youtube.com/watch?v=nRgxYX2Ve9w

These will define your biceps and also give your lower arms a work out, helping to stabilize elbows and wrists. This is especially important if you have rheumatoid arthritis.

- Start from a standing position with the weights resting on your thighs, palms facing down, backs of the forearms facing outwards.

- Lift the weights to shoulder height by using the elbows as a hinge.

- Release back down to first position. Press lightly as you go down to give your forearms even more of a work out.

- Repeat Steps 7 more times for 1 set of 8 to start with.

- Gradually increase the number of reps and sets at a comfortable pace as you continue to work out over the coming weeks. Increase to a higher weight once you no longer feel a real burn in your arms after 3 sets of 12 to 16 repetitions.

    Lateral raises
    https://www.youtube.com/watch?v=3VcKaXpzqRo

Lateral raises will work both biceps and triceps, plus your core as well.

- Start standing with the weights resting naturally at your sides, palms facing your sides.

- Raise the weights up to shoulder level so your arms are straight, elbows slightly relaxed, like a bird soaring.

- Hold in the upwards position, making a cross with your body.

- Slowly release the weights back down to the starting position.

- Repeat Steps for your desired number of reps and sets.

Note: Aim for a controlled lift both up and down, not arms flapping like a bird or flopping back down. To challenge yourself even more, try this as a slow lift. But beware of too heavy a load.

Lateral to overhead raises
https://www.youtube.com/watch?v=hUvTDZy_DBs

This exercise will work arms and shoulders, plus back and core. Do it on its own, or as the third and fourth moves to add to the previous exercise of lateral raises

- From the standing position, start with your arms extended outwards, elbows slightly bent, wrists upwards towards the sky.

- Raise the weights over your head by bring your upper arms close to your ears. Do not lock your elbows.

- Hold for a moment and slowly release back down to the starting position.

- Repeat 7 times for your first set.

Note: If combining with the previous exercise, use a rhythm similar to 3-step jumping jack. Start with weights at your side, lift laterally to shoulder height, then lift the weights overhead. Return back to the starting lower position using a count of three as well, overhead, down to shoulders and back down to sides.

2.) *Chest and Shoulders*

Pull up

https://www.youtube.com/watch?v=mRznU6pzez0

You should feel this exercise in your chest, shoulder, arms, back and waist.

- From the standing position, begin with your weights resting at about hip height, in front of your body and parallel to it, your inner wrists close to the tops of your thighs.

- Bend your elbows to bring the weights up to chin and shoulder height, upper arms in a fairly straight line from the shoulders to the elbows.

- Hold for 2 seconds

- Release in a smooth and controlled manner back down to first position.

Note: Do not lean forward or backwards when you do this in order to protect your lower back.

Gorilla lift

This exercise works chest, arms, shoulders and the sides of your torso to strengthen your core muscles and improve stability.

- From the standing position, begin with your weights resting at about hip height, slightly in front of your body with your inner wrists close to the tops of your thighs.

- Twist the weights slightly so they clear the sides of your body as your bring them upwards as if you were trying to tuck them your under your armpits.

- Bring up the weights along your side as far as they will go. Think of a gorilla or monkey scratching itself.

- Hold for a couple of seconds and then slowly release back down to the starting position.

- Repeat all steps paying particular attention to your form. Do not slouch - keep your hips firmly under you and over your feet.

Chest presses
https://www.youtube.com/watch?v=VmB1G1K7v94

Chest presses work biceps and triceps and can also improve your chest muscles. Men should develop good pectoral muscles (pecs) and women a higher, firmer bust line with this exercise.

- From standing, start with your elbows bent, weights at about shoulder level.

- Press your elbows together to meet in the center of your body at about shoulder level, in front of your face.

- As you switch between the first two steps, don't just move your elbows. Feel the muscles in your chest just under your arms working to press the weights together.

- Return to position first movement and repeat as many times as you wish to complete 1 set.

Notes: Be sure to maintain control over the weights in both directions. Keep your elbows at upper chest level rather than allowing the elbows to drop down towards your waist. In this way you can work all of the muscles deeply.

Keep your back straight-do not lean forward or backwards so you can protect your lower back muscles and give your chest a good work out. Press your inner forearms together to keep the weights at the same distance away from your body so you do not hit yourself in the face with the weights when you bring them to the center of your chest.

3.) *Core Strength, Arms and Legs*

Your core is the most important set of muscles in your body because they support all of the other muscle groups, such as your back, shoulders, arms and legs. A strong core means a strong back, leaving you less prone to lower back pain or injury.

Overhead lift
https://www.youtube.com/watch?v=UUBd9X7aHSI

Overhead lifts help improve all the muscles in your body, including arms and abs if you pay attention to your form when you are lifting. Just holding the weights over your head without moving to the next position will build muscle and bone.

- Start with your weights at about shoulder level, feet firmly planted, slightly apart.

- Push up by straightening your elbows until they are just about locked.

- Return to position in a controlled manner.

- Repeat 7 times for 1 set.

Notes: Be sure to maintain control over the weights in both directions so you do not smack yourself in the shoulder or drop your weights.

Keep the elbows at upper chest level in the downward position instead of dropping them towards your waist to work your arms and shoulders fully. Keep your back straight with your hips squarely over your feet. Do not lean forward or back to avoid back injury.

Overhead pull down

https://www.youtube.com/watch?v=qEwKCR5JCog

This will work out your shoulders, neck and chest muscles - just like the fancy cable machines at the gym. Focus on keeping control of the weights as you move from one position to the next to get your most effective work out.

- Start with your arms up over your head, weights touching.

- Pull the weights down slowly towards your shoulders by bending your elbows.

- As you pull down in a controlled manner, smoothly and without jerking, you should feel the muscles in your shoulders, abs, and the middle of your back being worked, not just in your upper arms and shoulders, for a stronger core.

- Return to the first position and repeat 7 more times to complete 1 set.

Note: To work shoulders, arms and core even more deeply, bring the weights to shoulder height but also lower your elbows as far down as they can go so they are tucked in against your sides around the level of your lower ribs.

Squat Lift

https://www.youtube.com/watch?v=oiEQ72KSQq4

Squats are a proven way to work out your abs, buttock and thighs. Combine them with weights and you soon see a difference in your muscle tone and overall appearance.

- Start with your weights in front of you at hip level, feet spread apart, hips squarely over them so your back is straight.

- Bend your knees as if you were going to sit down in a chair, still maintaining a straight rather than curved back and bringing the weights down to upper thigh level, in between your legs to keep your balance.

- Stand up straight again in a controlled manner, without locking the knees or jerking the weights upwards.

- Repeat steps seven more times to complete 1 set.

Note: Only bend the knees as much as you can without causing discomfort. Keep the weights in front of you so you do not lose your balance, but do not round your shoulders or hunch over. Keep your weight on your heels, not the toes of your foot.

Tricep kickbacks with squat

https://www.youtube.com/watch?v=m9me06UBPKc

Tricep kickbacks are an excellent focused exercise to improve the tone of the backs of your upper arms and shoulders. Adding it to a squat works all parts of your body, including your core. In this exercise you will be working one arm at a time.

- Start with your right arm.

- Lift one weight to tuck it up near your underarm, elbow bent.

- Bend your knees slightly into a squat as though you were going to sit down in a chair.

- Keep your back straight, not arched forward.

- Place your left hand on your left knee to steady you.

- Straighten your elbow so your arm stretches out backwards to its full extent.

- Do at least 8 repetitions per set.

- Repeat steps with your left arm.

Note: Keep your weight back to the heel. You should be able to wiggle your toes because the pressure is off the front of the foot. This releases pressure on the knees

4.) Legs

Lift and lunge

https://www.youtube.com/watch?v=rSvAMBGbQAY

Lunges, like squats, are effective in building core muscles and all of the muscles in your buttocks, thighs and calves. If you have any knee or ankle problems, or balance issues, start slowly and do not go too deeply or step out too widely. Also make sure you are wearing supportive sneakers and working out on a smooth, level surface that is not slippery.

- Begin with the weights relaxed at your sides at about hip height, with your feet close together.

- Working out the right side first, separate your feet to step sideways so you are in more of a sitting position.

- Hold the weights in front of you to keep your balance as you lunge. Do not step out too far or you might fall down. Do not lunge too far if you have any knee issues.

- To return to the starting position, you have two choices. Either step your right foot back to rest close to your left again, OR bring your left foot together with your right foot so you are walking sideways like a crab.

Variations of the last two motions will each work different muscles in your legs and the sides of your hips, which can all improve your balance and stability.

Repeat steps, this time starting with your left foot. Alternate right and left, or do 8 on each side. Vary it if you wish to make sure you do not get bored with your workout routine.

Note: Keep your weight back to the heel. You should be able to wiggle your toes because the pressure is off the front of the foot. This releases pressure on the knees.

Side extensions

https://www.youtube.com/watch?v=-AVmdPFIb7o

This is the first of three exercises for your legs that can be done with ankle weights. Follow your manufacturer's instructions on how to put them on safely.

This exercise work your inner thigh muscles and the hip flexors, which give you stability when you stand up or walk. Use a wall, countertop or sturdy chair that will not slide around on the floor to steady yourself while you work out. Work one side of the body at a time.

- Start with both your feet together on the floor, holding onto your wall, countertop or chair for balance.

- Using your right leg, extend it outwards so your legs are separated but your right foot is not touching the floor. Do not overextend or you could pull a muscle.

- Return to start position and repeat. Start with 1 set of 8 or 10 and work your way up.

- Try to control the leg up and down so you are not swinging the leg or kicking it out wildly.

- Repeat steps with your left leg.

Backwards extensions
https://www.youtube.com/watch?v=XP5HIlce8hA

This works your glutes, the muscles in your buttocks, and your legs. Use a countertop or sturdy chair that will not slide around on the floor to steady yourself while you work out. Work one side of the body at a time. Extend backwards slightly until you develop more strength in order to avoid injury.

- Start with both your feet together on the floor, holding onto your countertop or chair for balance.

- Beginning with your right leg, bend it at the knee.

- Leading with the knee and foot, extend the leg out behind you and away from the other leg until you feel a gentle pull going up the back of your leg to your buttock. Do not overextend or you could pull a muscle. Even small movements will work the muscle efficiently.

- Return to the starting position and repeat. Start with 1 set of 8 or 10 reps and gradually increase.

- Try to control the leg back and forth so your foot does not drop and you do not end up swinging your leg or kicking it out wildly.

- Repeat with your left leg.

Hip and leg extension
https://www.youtube.com/watch?v=e2T9VdGBofs

For this exercise, you will need to lie down on the floor on your side. This works your inner thigh muscles for toned and firm legs.

- Lie down on the floor on your right side to start with, legs straight out and in line with your body, which should also be straight. You can rest your head on your shoulder or propped up on your elbow and hand if you wish.

- Bend your left knee and bring that leg over your right one, which should still be straight along the floor. Find a comfortable position for the left leg, with the knee on the floor but not too far forward because that would twist the body too much.

- Flex the heel of your right foot so the toes are not pointing.

- Lift the right foot and leg off the floor, leading with the side of heel, which should be moving straight up towards the ceiling. Do not overstretch. Small movements are enough to work this set of muscles.

- Lower the right leg back down in a controlled manner.

- Repeat steps for a total of 8 in this set.

- Repeat steps with your left side. Lie on your left side, cross your right knee over, and lift your left leg off the floor, leading with your left heel.

Note: You can keep the hand not supporting your head on the floor in front of you to keep your balance. This will also prevent your hips from rolling back, which could lead to twisting and a back injury.

Once you finish all of the exercises you wish to do in one session, cool down with some stretches and shake out the muscles. Well done!

In this chapter, you have learned the following exercises

1) Arms
- Bicep curls
- Reverse bicep curls
- Lateral raises
- Lateral to overhead raises

2) Chest and Shoulders
- Pull up
- Gorilla lift
- Chest presses

3) Core Strength

- Overhead lift
- Overhead pull down
- Squat Lift
- Tricep kickbacks with squat

4) Legs
- Lift and lunge
- Side extensions
- Backward extensions
- Hip and leg extensions

Use these exercises one at a time, one set each, in rotation to work all parts of your body to build lean muscles that will improve your appearance. That is, work arms, then core or legs, the shoulders and chest, then back to arms and so on.

Start slowly and gradually work your way up to more repetitions and 3 sets. Then go up to a higher weight to continue building muscle. Remember, toned and trim muscles will not only make you look great, but will also help you burn even more calories.

Conclusion

So there you have it, the many reasons why light weights are so good for your fitness and overall well-being, plus a range of exercises to help you get started. Light weights offer a range of health benefits all in the comfort of your own home. You can use them standing up, lying down, or sitting. You can use them for a whole body work out, or improve your appearance toning flabby arms or weak legs.

For your upper body, you do not need a lot of expensive equipment to get started. Use cans and bottles from your pantry or laundry room to start lifting light weights. Once you need to increase the weights gradually, then you can consider buying a set of weights or Aquabells, dumbbells, and/or resistance bands. A set of ankle weights can help you tone your legs even more rapidly than just using your own body weight.

Start slowly, putting safety first. Pay attention to your form, not tilting your hips forwards or backwards. Lift the weights in a smooth, steady motion without jerking. Begin with 1 set of 8-10 repetitions to a count that is comfortable for you. Alternate between arms, legs and abs so you do not overwork any one given set of muscles.

Light weights can help you slim down and tone up as long as you stick to a regular workout routine of lifting at least twice a week, not every day because your muscles need to rest for 24 to 48 hours after your workout.

Alternate with cardio activities on the days you are not strength training and see what a difference your work outs can make to your health and appearance, for a fitter and more attractive new you.

Resources

Harvard Health Beat - 5 of the best exercises you can ever do

http://www.health.harvard.edu/staying-healthy/5-of-the-best-exercises-you-can-ever-do

Sharecare - Improve Your Balance

https://www.sharecare.com/health/fitness-exercise/article/improve-your-balance

Exercises to Improve Your Balance and Reduce the Risk of a Fall

http://www.mccn.edu/library/patienteducation/duplicatenetitp_/patienteducatio_/exerciseandreha_/exercises_/exercisestoimpr/ExercisestoImproveYourBalanceandReducetheRiskofaFall.pdf

Mobility Decline in Old Age

Exercise and Sports Sciences Reviews 2013;41(1):19-25.

http://www.medscape.com/viewarticle/777551_6

Helping Seniors with Chronic Illness Improve Their Quality of Life

http://www.lifelinesys.com/content/blog/healthcare-professionals/successful-aging-strategies/helping-seniors-with-chronic-illness-improve-their-quality-of-life

Bone density sharply enhanced by weight training, even in the elderly

http://www.naturalnews.com/010528_bone_density_mineral.html

What is metabolic syndrome?

http://www.nhlbi.nih.gov/health/health-topics/topics/ms

Definition of Metabolic Syndrome

http://circ.ahajournals.org/content/109/3/433.full

10 ways to boost your metabolism

http://www.webmd.com/diet/ss/slideshow-boost-your-metabolism

The Top Ten Ways to Decrease Elevated Triglycerides

https://www.umassmed.edu/uploadedfiles/LoweringTriglycerides.pdf

Aquabells Hand Weights

http://amzn.to/1VLCAd5

Tone Fitness Dumbbell Set, 20 pounds, 2, 3 and 5 pound pairs of weights

http://amzn.to/21sF3js

Tone Fitness Dumbbell Set, 32 pounds, 3, 5 and 8 pound pairs of weights

http://amzn.to/210pE4o

Crown Sporting Goods Set, 30 pounds, 3 5 and 7 pound weights

http://amzn.to/21xNmHi

Weider Ankle Weights, 5 lbs each

http://amzn.to/1LKxqs0

Other Senior Health and Fitness Books by This Author

If you would like to read more about Senior Health and Fitness, here is a list of the <u>titles, CreateSpace links and descriptions:</u>

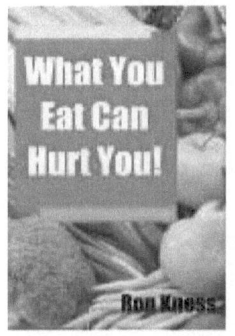

<u>What You Eat Can Hurt You</u>

https://www.createspace.com/4963196

Do you know that certain foods increase your risk for inflammation, disease and illness? It's true! And certain foods can help cure and heal you if you do get sick. Knowing which foods to eat and which ones to avoid empowers you to manage your own health.

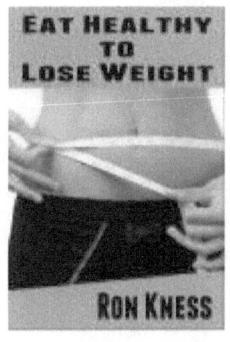

<u>Eat Healthy to Lose Weight</u>

https://www.createspace.com/4962939

As you read through our book, we show you which foods you should and should not be eating to reach your weight loss goal, along with discussing how to maintain your weight loss and stay within a few pounds of your goal weight. Banish the weight you keep gaining back each time by learning how to live a healthy lifestyle.

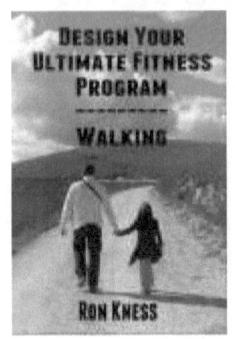

Design Your Ultimate Fitness Program -
Walking

https://www.createspace.com/5252272

In my book Design Your Ultimate Fitness
Program – Walking, we discuss the
considerations that need to be made when
designing a custom walking program, along
with:
• Equipment needed
• Wearable technology you can use to track your walking
• And how to make walking more challenging

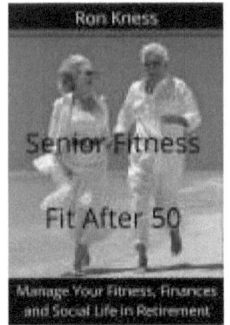

Senior Fitness – Fit After 50: Learn How to
Manage Your Fitness, Finances and Social Life
in Retirement

https://www.createspace.com/5474751

Inside you will discover answers to your most
pressing questions:
• What do I need to know about downsizing my
home?
• What are the best tips for staying healthy as you approach your
50's?
• When should I start planning for retirement?
• I am worried about being lonely once I retire, do others feel the
same?
• Is it worthwhile to carry two homes during retirement?
And more…

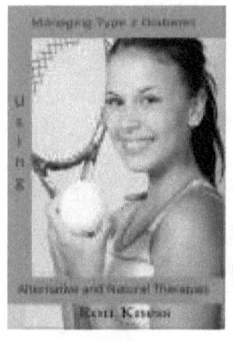

Managing Type 2 Diabetes Using Alternative And Natural Therapies

https://www.createspace.com/5401244

While Type 2 diabetes can be managed medically, there are many alternative natural and holistic methods of therapy and treatment that can further enhance quality of life and minimize the effects of this disease. In this book, I discuss 12 different types, including yoga, reflexology and acupuncture to name just three.

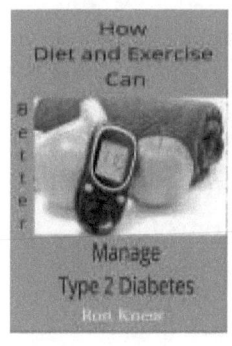

How Diet and Exercise Can Better Manage Type 2 Diabetes

https://www.createspace.com/5404845

Of the different types of diabetes, only Type 2 can be reversed. In my book How Diet and Exercise Can Better Manage Type 2 Diabetes, we reveal the three things you can do to best manage your disease, including:
• Diet
• Exercise
• Weight management

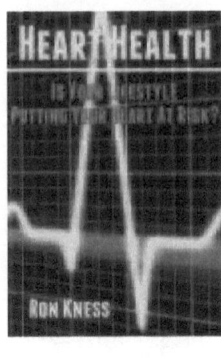

Heart Health: Is Your Lifestyle Putting Your Heart at Risk?

https://www.createspace.com/5464020

In my ebook Is Your Lifestyle Putting Your Heart At Risk? we discuss the six greatest risks to your heart and the lifestyle changes you can make to mitigate them.

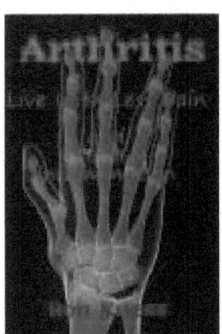

Arthritis – Live Wth Less Pain and Inflammation: Tips and Techniques You Can Use to Lessen the Pain and Inflammation

https://www.createspace.com/5457441

Discover Simple Tips & Information That Will Help Reduce The Painful Symptoms Of Arthritis!

You learn things like:
• Simple and effective information that will help you manage the pain and inflammation that comes along with arthritis, so that you can live an active, full life without debilitating pain.
• The different types of arthritis, their symptoms and how to alleviate their painful side effects.
• The pros and cons of over-the-counter arthritis medications, plus simple tips that will help you know how to choose the right supplements.
• Free, yet effective ways to get relief from arthritis pain and inflammation, so you don't have to suffer anymore.

the effects arthritis can have significant impact on your physical and mental well-being, but this books shows you how to overcome its painful symptoms and live life relatively pain free.

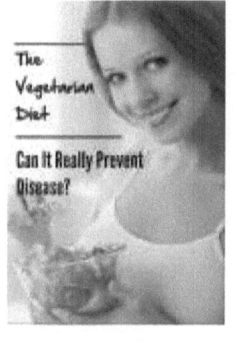

The Vegetarian Diet – Can It Really Prevent Disease?

https://www.createspace.com/5519874

Is a vegetarian diet right for you? Multiple studies have shown over and over that a vegetarian diet goes along way in preventing certain chronic diseases, such as:

• Heart Disease
• Cancer
• Diverticulitis
• Type 2 Diabetes
• Hypertension
• Obesity
• Kidney Failure

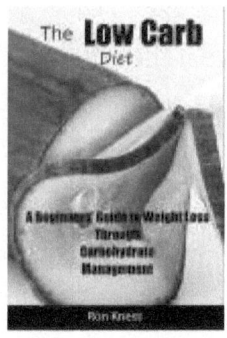

The Low Carb Diet: A Beginner's Guide to Weight Loss Through Carbohydrate Management

https://www.createspace.com/5416348

In my book "The Low-Carb Diet – A Beginners' Guide to Weight Loss Through Carbohydrate Management", I reveal a successful method of losing weight based in part on the amount and type of carbohydrates you consume.

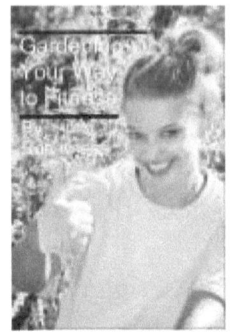

Gardening Your Way to Fitness: The Fun Way to Get Fit and Provide Beauty and Healthful Bounty for Your Family

https://www.createspace.com/5459564

The gym is a great place to stay fit during the colder seasons, but once the temperature turns warmer you want to spend more time outside. Plus, you'll have the benefit of fresh wholesome produce to enjoy by growing vegetables in your backyard garden.

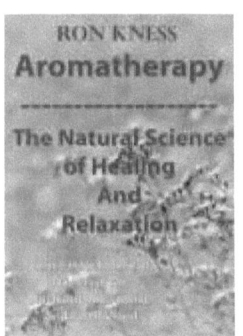

Aromatherapy - The Science of Healing and Relaxation: Learn How Essential Oils Elicit The Relaxation Response And Alter Mood

https://www.createspace.com/5714434

In my book Aromatherapy – The Science of Healing and Relaxation, we reveal the natural holistics methods you can use to heal the body from certain medical issues and to relive stress through relaxation. In particular we talk about:
• Aromatherapy - what it is and how it works
• Essential Oils – how the effects of certain aromas differs from others
• Recipes – how to make your own essential oil combinations

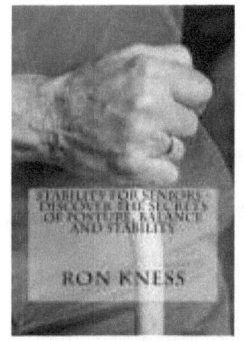

Stability for Seniors: Discover the Secrets of Posture, Balance and Stability

https://www.createspace.com/6096479

Many people sacrifice their health in pursuit of their career. They are so busy making a living that they neglect to make a life. The excuse that they do not have time to exercise is tossed about so frequently that they end up letting their health and fitness slide.

If you are not regularly active, you will have muscular atrophy over time. Your flexibility will decrease. Your core strength will diminish. As time progresses, you will be less limber and more rigid.

This is exactly how people age poorly. It's a process that has snowballed over time.

Only with regular exercise and a healthy diet can you have a body that is fit and has the ability to almost reverse aging.

If you have neglected your health for years and life seems to be a chore now because you can't get around without assistance, do not feel dejected.

You can remedy the situation. You can restore the strength, balance and stamina that you have lost. It is never too late to become what you might have been.

This guide will show you exactly what you need to do to restore your balance, strengthen your core and give you the ability to live life to its fullest. Read how …

About the Author

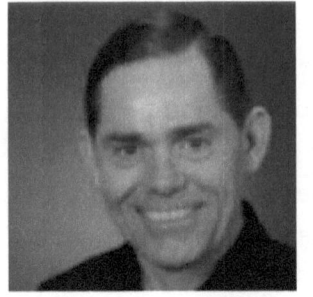

I grew up in Central Minnesota, where my parents own and operated a fishing resort. Once out of high school I tried a couple of semesters of college, only to quit halfway through the Spring term; I decided at that time that college wasn't for me.

Then I decided to follow my father's previous occupation as an auto mechanic. I graduated from a two-year of vocational training course and worked as a mechanic. While in vocational training, I decided to join the National Guard where I eventually ended up working full-time for 32 years.

So how does all of this relate to writing? In one of my leadership schools, the instructor, who was an English teacher at a juvenile detention center, presented writing to me in a whole new way - a way that started to develop my interest in working with words.

Fast forward about 40 years and I now have over 50 books listed on Amazon for Kindle and CreateSpace.

www.ingramcontent.com/pod-product-compliance
Lightning Source LLC
Chambersburg PA
CBHW030533290526
45786CB00004B/1702